FOODS FOR A HEALTHY LIFESTYLE

Cooking Instructions

By

Elizabeth D. Lewis

TABLE OF CONTENTS

INTRODUCTION

Parents who want to learn how to cook in order to live a healthy lifestyle are the target audience for this book. Healthy living does not include a fast remedy. It is a journey that started with our conception and continues till we breathe our last. Therefore, the journey to our well-being will call for long-distance training.

Adopting a long-term perspective on your well-being makes it easier to handle making little improvements. When you realize that a challenge is only a new turn in your health, you won't feel as frightened by setbacks and health issues along the trip. It is usual for your body to change through time; it may just want a certain kind of TLC from you to keep thriving.

Your body contains many billions of cells, and each one has a specific structure and function. How well you treat your cells will determine how well you will feel. In this book, I'll go through how to keep fit and conduct yourself appropriately. First, we'll talk about the nutrients your Body needs to be healthy. Sugar is used by the food business to make people dependent on its products.

Conventionally raised cattle, as well as conventionally farmed food, may be harmful to both people and the environment. In contrast to what was formerly believed, naturally occurring animal and plant lipids are advantageous.

Sweeteners and sugar may make you obese and possibly be harmful. Starches and grains provide slight improvement. In general, milk and other dairy products are harmful to adult humans.

Non-starchy vegetables should make up more than half of your plate, and just a little quantity of animal protein should be consumed at one time. These meals must be raw and free of hormones, pesticides, and insecticides.

Supplements, herbs, and nutrient-rich spices should be used to bolster people's diets.

CHAPTER 1

PRINCIPLES OF NUTRITION

An organism utilizes food to sustain its existence via a biochemical and physiological process known as nutrition. It gives living things nutrition that can be processed to produce energy and chemical building blocks. The nutrients that come from the food we consume are substances that the body utilizes for constructing and mending tissues,
giving heat and energy, defending the body against sickness, and
assisting in the removal of waste products from the system.

Sources of Nutrients

There are six fundamental nutrients, namely: carbs, proteins, lipids, mineral stuff, vitamins, and water.

Carbohydrates

The body's primary energy source is carbohydrate-based. They are the dietary fiber, sugars, and carbohydrates found in dairy and plant-based diets. Plant-based foods are the main sources of carbohydrates. They may also be found in dairy products such as lactose, a milk sugar. Bread, pasta, potatoes, rice, and cereals are examples of foods high in carbohydrates. In living things, carbohydrates play several functions, including providing energy. Carbohydrate byproducts have a role in the immune system, the onset of disease, blood clotting, and reproductive processes. Saccharides usually referred to as carbohydrates or sugars, are the body's primary source of energy. Carbohydrates provide 4 calories per gram.

Glucose, produced by the body's breakdown of carbohydrates, serves as the main fuel for the brain and muscles.

One of the three macronutrients—nutrients that the body needs in more significant quantities—is carbohydrates. There are many different types of

carbohydrates in the food, including the following:
A kind of carbohydrate that the body finds difficult to digest is dietary fiber. Fruits, vegetables, nuts, seeds, beans, and whole grains all naturally contain it.
Total sugars comprise both added sugars, which are often found in baked goods, sweets, and desserts, as well as sugars that are present naturally in meals, such as dairy products. Sugars are readily absorbed and digested by the body.
A form of carbohydrate that the body can not completely digest is sugar alcohol. They taste sweet and have fewer calories than sugar. In foods like chewing gum, baked goods, and confectionery, sugar alcohols are used as low-calorie sweeteners.

Protein

Large, intricate molecules known as proteins serve a variety of vital functions in the body. They are crucial for the construction, operation, and control of the body's tissues and organs and carry out the majority of their job within cells. Protein is found in practically every organ, tissue, and bodily part of the body, including muscle, bone, skin, and hair. It is responsible for creating the hemoglobin that carries oxygen in your blood as well as the enzymes that power various chemical processes. At least 10,000 distinct proteins make up you, and they maintain you that way. Protein is an essential part of any diet. Depending on a person's age and sex, different quantities of protein are required. Protein is one of the three macronutrients—nutrients the body needs in more significant quantities. Fat and carbohydrates are the other macronutrients.

Proteins are made up of long strands of amino acids. There are twenty amino acids. The particular amino acid sequence used in a protein determines both its structure and intended application.

The 20 amino acids required by the body to produce protein are alanine, arginine, asparagine, aspartic acid, cysteine, glutamic acid, glutamine, glycine, histidine, isoleucine,

leucine, lysine, methionine, phenylalanine, proline, serine, threonine, tryptophan, tyrosine, and valine.

The human body does not produce nine essential amino acids, hence they must be obtained through diet. The nine amino acids recognized as crucial are histidine, isoleucine, leucine, lysine, methionine, phenylalanine, threonine, tryptophan, and valine. All necessary amino acids must be present in a protein for it to be considered complete; otherwise, it lacks one or more of these amino acids. Animal products, quinoa, and soy all have complete proteins.

Incomplete proteins are those that don't contain all the required amino acids. The vast majority of plant foods that include incomplete proteins include beans, nuts, and grains.

Incomplete protein sources may be combined to provide a meal that contains all nine required amino acids. Examples include peanut butter on whole wheat toast or rice and beans.

What does protein do in the body?

Protein is involved in a variety of body functions, such as

blood coagulation,

fluid balance, and

immune system reactions.

vision

hormones

enzyme

Particularly throughout infancy, adolescence, and pregnancy, protein is crucial for growth and development.

Sources of Protein

Foods from both animals and plants may be great providers of protein. The following foods are classified as protein foods by the guidelines:

seafood

poultry eggs and lean meats

Beans, peas, nuts, and seeds are examples of legumes.

soy-based goods

Milk, cheese, and yogurt are dairy products that also include protein. Although often less than other sources, whole grains and veggies do contain some protein.

People who follow a vegetarian or vegan diet may need to arrange their meals to make sure they satisfy their protein demands since animal items often contain larger levels of protein than plant foods.

Fat

Fat may be defined as any ester of fatty acids or a mixture. Food and living creatures include these chemicals most often. Fat is an essential macronutrient. There are several types of dietary fat, some of which are much healthier than others. Fat is essential for numerous bodily functions. Both the nerves and the bones are shielded and it provides energy. The actions of other nutrients are also made possible by fat. However, not all dietary lipid benefits are equal: The risk of sickness is decreased by monounsaturated and polyunsaturated fats, sometimes known as "healthy" unsaturated fats. Among the foods high in healthful fats include

Fish, nuts, seeds, and vegetable oils (such as canola, olive, sunflower, and maize oils).
Trans fats, for example, increase the risk of getting a disease even in little quantities. The majority of trans fats are produced by partially hydrogenated oil and are present in processed foods. Many of these products thankfully no longer contain trans fats.
Saturated fats nevertheless have a negative impact on health and are best consumed in moderation, while being less hazardous than trans fats. Some examples of foods rich in saturated fat are red meat, butter, cheese, and ice cream. In certain plant-based fats, such as coconut and palm oils, saturated fats are also present.
Foods including meat, dairy, snacks, and baked goods may include saturated and trans fats. Foods that include unsaturated, healthful fats include nuts, seeds, oils, and avocados.

Vitamins

Organic substances known as vitamins are virtually ever found in natural foods. A vitamin shortage may increase the risk of developing certain health issues. Since the vitamin is an organic substance, carbon must be present. Additionally, it is a nutrient that the body may need food to provide.

There are now 13 recognized vitamins.

water-soluble and fat-soluble vitamins

Vitamins may dissolve in either fat or water or both. Below, we discuss both kinds:

Vitamins soluble in fat

The fat-soluble vitamins A, D, E, and K are. Fat-soluble vitamins are stored by the body in fatty tissue in the liver, where they may remain for days or even months at a time.

Dietary fats facilitate the intestinal absorption of fat-soluble vitamins by the organism.

water-soluble nutrients

Vitamins that are water-soluble pass through the body quickly and cannot be stored. Through urination, they exit the body. People need a more consistent supply of water-soluble vitamins than fat-soluble ones as a result. All of the B vitamins, including vitamin C, are water-soluble.

Minerals

Our bodies need minerals for optimal growth and development; they may be found in food and the soil. In order to carry out crucial life-sustaining activities, organisms need the chemical element known as a mineral as an essential nutrient. However, lists of the main vitamins, minerals, and the four structural elements that make up the human body—oxygen, hydrogen, carbon, and nitrogen—frequently exclude these elements by weight (nitrogen is considered a "mineral" for plants, as it often is included in fertilizers). These four components make up around 96% of the weight of the human body, with huge minerals (macrominerals) and minor minerals making up the remaining 4%. (also known as trace elements).

Nutrient minerals cannot be created biochemically by living beings since they are elements. Plants get minerals from the soil. The bulk of the minerals that humans consume come from eating plants and animals as well as from drinking water. Along with essential vitamins, essential fatty acids, and essential amino acids, minerals are one of the four categories of essential nutrients. The five primary minerals in the human body are magnesium, calcium, phosphorus, potassium, and sodium. All of the components that are still found in a human body are referred to as "trace elements." Sulfur, iron, chlorine, copper, zinc, manganese, molybdenum, iodine, selenium, and other trace elements all have specific metabolic functions in the human body.

Simple compounds are the most common kind of chemical that organisms eat. Plants absorb the dissolved components from the soil, which move up the food chain by being eaten by herbivores and omnivores. Larger species may also consume soil (geophagia) or use mineral resources, such as salt licks, to get limited minerals that are not accessible via other food sources.

Bacteria and fungi must weather fundamental components in order to release nutrients for both their own nutrition and the nutrition of other species in the ecological food chain. Mammals can only use one element, cobalt, once bacteria have converted it into complex molecules (like vitamin B12). Minerals are used by both animals and bacteria in the biomineralization process, which they utilize to create exoskeletons, mollusk shells, seashells, and bones.

Water

Water makes up almost two-thirds of the body. It is a component of every cell and tissue and is essential for managing biological processes. The amount of water in the body affects all of these activities, including digestion, absorption, temperature control, and waste removal.

Quick facts about water to drink

Human adults have 60% water, and 90% of our blood is water.

There is no set daily need for how much water should be drunk.

For the kidneys and other biological processes, water is crucial.

Dehydration may make the skin more prone to wrinkles and skin conditions.

Switching to water from soda may aid with weight reduction.

Advantages of water consumption

All of the body's cells and organs need water to operate correctly.

Our bodies need water for the following reasons:

The lubrication of the joints. Water makes up around 80% of cartilage, which is present in spinal disks and joints. Joint soreness may be brought on by a gradual decline in the joint's ability to absorb damage.

It produces saliva and mucus. Saliva assists in the digestion of meals and keep the lips, nose, and eyes moist. This prevents wear and friction. Drinking water helps keep the mouth healthy as well. When sweetened drinks are replaced, it may help reduce tooth decay.

It provides oxygen to the body. More than 90% of the water in the blood, which carries oxygen to different parts of the body, is salt water.

Improved skin quality and look. Dehydration may increase the skin's susceptibility to aging-related skin disorders.

It protects the spinal cord, brain, and other fragile tissues. Dehydration may affect the structure and operation of the brain. It also aids in the production of hormones and neurotransmitters. Dehydration over an extended period of time may interfere with judgment and thinking.
It manages the body's temperature. Water that has been stored in the middle layers of the skin comes to the surface as sweat when the body heats up. When it evaporates, the body becomes even colder. in a match. Some specialists believe that when a person's body is dehydrated, heat retention increases and heat stress tolerance diminishes. The physical strain may be lessened if you drink plenty of water if you experience heat stress while exercising.
The digestive system needs it. Water is needed by the stomach in order for it to operate properly. Dehydration may lead to constipation, excessively high stomach acid, and digestive problems. The likelihood of stomach ulcers and heartburn has increased as a consequence.

Waste from the body is flushed. Water is required for sweating, urination, and excrement disposal.

It aids in maintaining blood pressure. Lack of water may cause blood to thicken, which can increase blood pressure.

Flights need it. When a person is dehydrated, their body tries to stop water loss by constricting their airways. As a consequence, asthma and allergies may worsen.

It makes it easier to acquire minerals and nutrients. These decompose in water, enabling them to enter the body at different points.

It protects against kidney damage. The fluid balance of the body is managed by the kidneys. Lack of water consumption may lead to illnesses like kidney stones and other ailments.

It enhances exercise performance.

CHAPTER 2

MEAL PREPARATION

The meals we consume may be categorized into three main groups:

Foods like proteins that aid in the growth of muscle or meat.

Foods that provide you energy, such as carbohydrates and fats

Foods are rich in minerals and vitamins that are protective.

Meal planning must contain foods from these groups. Three meals a day are advised, with two being substantial and one being smaller. Breakfast is necessary for a successful start to the day's work. Every day, especially first thing in the morning, fruit should be ingested. Green vegetables provide salt and vitamins.

Promoting a daily intake of high-quality protein is necessary. Cereals and root vegetables are good sources of carbohydrates, although there are other options on the menu. You should eat some fat or oil each day. There should be enough supply of "protective" foods like milk and eggs. Promoting fresh meals is important. Choose seasonal foods whenever you can. A diverse diet is essential. Make a plan since it will save you money, time, and effort. Take the family's size into consideration. The meal to prepare depends on the population's age. Serve well-cooked, healthy, simplified meals. Make use of a range of serving utensils while presenting meals to the family.

Breakfast

The first meal of the day, breakfast is often eaten in the morning. a meal to break the previous night's fast. There are several "typical" or "traditional" breakfast meals, with food options differing globally based on areas and customs.

Suggestions for breakfast

Fruit: Fruits are a great source of fiber as well as important vitamins and minerals. It also offers a variety of antioxidants that are good for your health, including those found in pawpaw, oranges, pineapple, and fruit juice.

Oats, millet meal, rice water, cornmeal, and porridge are among the cereals.
Rice, plantains, bread, and root vegetables all contain carbs.
peppers and tomatoes are vegetables.
Fat: butter and margarine.
Meat and Fish
ingest milk, water, coffee, tea, etc.

Midday (lunch)

Lunch is a meal consumed at about noon. It is often eaten after breakfast as the second meal of the day. The size and personality will differ depending on the person and the family.

Dinner (supper)

The biggest and most formal meal of the day, known as dinner, is often served in the evening.

Ideas for lunch and supper

Meat, Fish, beans, and peas are all sources of protein.
Carbohydrates include plantains, grains, and root vegetables.

Fats include palm kernel, nut, and nut oil.
Vegetables: lettuce, cucumbers, tomatoes, boiling green vegetables, and salads.
Fruit: melons, oranges, and bananas.
Custards and fruit salad are sweets.

CHAPTER 3

FOOD COOKING

The practice of utilizing heat to prepare food for consumption is known as cooking. In order to represent local circumstances, cooking methods and ingredients vary greatly, from grilling meals over an open flame to utilizing electric burners to baking in a variety of ovens.

Food is cooked for the following reasons:

Easier to consume food as a result of cooking.

It enhances the flavor and palatability of meals.

Food is simpler to digest as a result.

It makes food safe to consume.

Food looks better after being cooked.

It enhances the flavor of meals.

Techniques for cooking

Food Preparation Using Dry Heat

When food is prepared with "dry heat," it is subjected to a source of intense heat that might come from below or above (and usually in an oven). Compared to "wet heat" cooking, this kind of heat raises food temperatures significantly. When cooking using dry heat, you may use less fat (such as oil or butter) and yet produce a lot of delicious food. When cooked with dry heat, meats, poultry, Fish, tofu, and vegetables are wonderful.

Using dry heat to cook is quite flexible.

Cooking using dry heat may be done in a variety of methods, including grilling, broiling, baking, roasting, sautéing or stir-frying, and searing:

Grilling

When grilling, the food is cooked using heat from below. A typical grilling method is barbecuing. To prevent food from sticking, use a hot grill, and cover the pan to cook food rapidly. Grill beef steaks or hamburgers made with ground beef, salmon, or seasoned chicken breasts. The grill is a great way to cook kebabs that include both meat and veggies or vegetables and tofu. Try some of these tasty and nutritious grilling dish ideas. You can still grill meals if you don't have a barbecue by utilizing an indoor grill, a griddle, or a grill pan on your cooktop (like a sandwich maker).

Broiling

Similar to grilling, but using oven heat from above, is broiling (instead of below). Because it is only exposed to very high heat for a brief period while being broiled, food cooks fast and evenly. Put your meal on the top rack of your oven and turn the oven on to broil. In a toaster oven, food may also be broiled. Simply keep an eye on your meal since it will heat up rapidly. Similar to grilling, broiling is a great method for many types of meat, including loin or chops of beef, lamb, or hog. Try seafood like this delicious Tandoori haddock or chicken parts like the thighs, breasts, or legs. Broiling may also be used to cook vegetables, such as these thyme-braised mushrooms.

Baking

Similar to broiling in the oven, baking also involves surrounding the food with heat. The movement of air within the oven bakes the food.

The slowest way of cooking using dry heat is baking. You could see that food bakes more quickly if you have a convection oven. This occurs as a result of additional fans being used to move the heated air within the oven. For meat recipes like these Green Meatballs, baking works nicely. Like this Mediterranean-baked Fish, Fish bakes wonderfully when covered with fresh veggies and herbs.

Roasting

Typically, food is roasted in an oven where the dry heat can circulate and cook the meal evenly. To get a crisp, browned top, roasting often starts at a higher temperature than baking does. Reduce the heat after a brown surface has developed until the meal has cooked to a safe internal temperature, which you can check with a food thermometer. Roast beef, such as prime rib, whole or cut-up chicken parts, and pork, such as this, are often prepared by roasting. Pork Tenderloin with Glazed Carrots and similar veggies fried parmesan carrots

With dry heat, cooking is made simple.

maintain high temperatures. Before adding food to the grill during cooking, ensure sure the grates are hot. Make sure the oil is just below the smoking point while sautéing or stirring-frying. The fat or oil you are using reaches its smoking point when it begins to emit smoke or an unpleasant odor. Avoid heating a fat over its smoke point since doing so may alter the fat's flavor and nutritional value.

Maintain precise temperatures. The actual temperature inside your oven and the setting you set it to are often two different things. To determine the actual temperature of the oven, place an oven thermometer in the center.

Preserve airflow. To help the food cook evenly both inside and out while roasting, set the entire chicken or beef roast on top of a bed of vegetables or a roasting rack.

Make careful you roast your meal rather than steam it! Avoid using a lid and use a shallow baking sheet or roasting pan. This promotes airflow without generating steam.

Use better oil for cooking. Because they don't burn as quickly as naturally solid fats like butter, go for healthy unsaturated fats like canola or safflower oil.

Foods Cooked Using Wet Heat.

Wet heat may be used to cook in a variety of ways.

The many wet heat cooking techniques include braising, boiling, steaming, poaching, and simmering.

Braising

Braising is a fantastic method for preparing flavorful but difficult foods. Raising is accomplished in two phases. Firstly, brown food using dry heat. To make it softer, add a little liquid and cook it gently. The food is cooked gradually by the liquid, generating rich flavor and softening fibrous food. Foods should be prepared until they are "fork-tender," or easily pierced with a fork. For less-priced meat or vegetable cuts, braising is a great method. Use this technique for making Moroccan lamb tagine.

Boiling

Boiling food is often associated with being overdone and lacking in nourishment. However, boiling is a speedier method of cooking food than dry heat and may be preferred in certain circumstances. It's crucial to cook food at a full boil while boiling it. As a result, the liquid should be rapidly creating plenty of large bubbles. For dishes including legumes, such as curry lentils, sweet potatoes, and cauliflower, try boiling.

Steaming

Food is cooked by steaming using moisture from a little quantity of simmering or boiling water. Avoid submerging food directly in the water while steaming it. Instead, set the meal over the liquid on a rack or in a steamer basket. To help keep the moisture within, cover the pot with a lid. To preserve the food's flavor, form, and texture, steaming is preferable to boiling or poaching. Steamed food also loses fewer nutrients than raw food. Any vegetable, including broccoli, carrots, and green beans, may be prepared simply and with little fat by steaming. Add freshly squeezed lemon juice after steaming your preferred veggies to enhance flavor.

More advice on using moist heat while cooking

Maintain a low temperature. Liquids must be maintained at a low temperature while braising, steaming, poaching, or boiling for gradual, even cooking to maximize flavor and softness.

Retain the moisture within. To retain the water within your pot, you need a tight-fitting cover. This wet heat cooks the meal.

Play around with various liquids. A fantastic method to flavor food is to poach it in juice, stock, or broth.

Pick the appropriate components. When braising, you don't need to purchase pricey cuts of meat. Cheaper cuts of meat work best since this technique of cooking softens food, providing it an affordable option to incorporate meat into your meals.

CHAPTER 4

RECIPES FOR ILL AND THE RECOVERING (CONVALESCENT)

One who is ill is invalid. A person who is convalescing is no longer unwell but is instead gradually recovering from their ailment. They both have very fragile intestines. Consequently, their foods must be simple to digest. They need a lot of protein, vitamins, and minerals in addition to energy-boosting meals. Although fat is a highly concentrated kind of energy, it is difficult to digest, thus it shouldn't be given to sick people or those recovering from an illness. It is essential to adopt cooking techniques that will make the meal simple to digest, such as stewing, steaming, and boiling.

Three types of ill diets may be distinguished: liquid, light, and convalescent or invalid diet.

Juice diet

The only food on a liquid diet is liquids, the most valued of which is milk. The beef, chicken, and mutton broths, the oyster and clam broth, the albumen water, the egg-nog, egg cream, the mulled wine, the tea, and the coffee are all superb. As the patient begins to recover, soft custards and jellies prepared with wine, lemon, coffee, or orange juice that rapidly turn into liquid when consumed may be added to this list. A liquid diet is prescribed when a patient suffers from a severe and hazardous disease. Typically, the doctor will recommend the quantity of food to be provided and the times at which it should be delivered.

Light diet

A light diet consists of all items permitted in a soft diet, whole-grain cereals, readily digestible raw fruits and vegetables, and raw dairy products. Foods aren't ground or pureed. Patients who don't need a soft diet but can't yet resume a complete diet might utilize this diet as an interim regimen.

Rehabilitation diet

The liquid and light diets and any readily digestible and nutrient-dense foods are all included in the convalescent's diet. Beef, mutton, and chicken may be served as meats together with the game, particularly venison, and birds, but never either hog or veal. They are challenging to absorb. All varieties of eggs, including soft-cooked, scrambled, poached, and omelets, as well as well-baked potatoes, creamed potatoes, celery, snow pudding, cream of rice pudding, and tapioca cream, as well as jellies made from both fruits and gelatin, Graham bread, Graham gems, rusk, and, really, any well-made bread, as well as good cake.

A recovering person should consume enough high-quality milk, chocolate, well-brewed tea and coffee, decent wine on occasion, and various drinking and mineral waters. Pastry, dark or poorly produced cakes, hog, veal, any strongly spiced meat dish cooked with gravy, all forms of fried food, sausages, heavy puddings, poorly made bread, lobsters, and crabs are a few things to stay away from.

Essential Guidelines for Providing Meals for Ill (Invalids and convalescents)

It is crucial to carefully follow the doctor's or dietician's directions if they have been consulted. Even when it is evident that the hospitalized patient cannot consume ordinary meals, the doctor or dietician is often not even contacted in situations of mild indisposition. Therapeutic diets are offered to them, such as fluid diets, light diets, and liquid diets.

A liquid diet should be maintained if there is an indication of fever, which is when the temperature is higher than usual. This should include milk, apple water, diluted blackcurrant juice, and liquid juices like orangeade or lemonade. These beverages have to be sweetened with glucose, which may be quickly absorbed into the bloodstream and so give energy to those who have indigestion. If the flavor is tolerable to the invalid, honey is virtually as quickly absorbed as glucose, providing diversity.

Vitamin C, which is included in fruit juices and aids in blood vessel health and clearing of the bloodstream, is provided. Fruit juices should be strained to eliminate any pulp, which may irritate the stomach lining, if there is a gastrointestinal condition present, such as an ulcer.

Fruit juices might be changed up by adding pepper soup, vegetable broth, or animal broth. Fruit-flavored beverages or broths are preferred by patients because they are more refreshing and thirst-quenching.

Milky beverages may be consumed in moderation unless a doctor or nutritionist advises against them. A patient should drink roughly 2 1/2 liters (5 pints) of fluids every day when they are experiencing a fever. Any liquid that remains in a sick room should be thrown away since it may serve as a breeding ground for bacteria.

During sickness, some strength is lost. By consuming foods that are simple to digest for bodybuilding, such as milk, eggs, white Fish, and chicken, this loss of power is recovered. These meals include calcium, a mineral that is essential for recuperation. If briefly cooked, such as in eggnog, the readily digestible protein foods in milk and eggs are also quickly assimilated.

Whitefish or fowl is the next item to be introduced after the patient can digest solid food. Don't eat greasy Fish.

Select appropriate cooking techniques, such as steaming, boiling, or baking. For the ill, avoid frying since the strong flavor is unpleasant and indigestible.

Use delicate meat for recovering patients since it is easily absorbed by the body.

Usually, a sick person has a bland appetite. Therefore, provide a range of delicious foods.

Small, regular meals should be provided and consumed five to six times daily.

The food should be properly served on clean, well-maintained serving trays that are big enough to facilitate easy eating.

Serve each patient's meal with a generous amount of garnish. It seems more alluring.

Meals must be adequately balanced when a patient has reached the late stage of recuperation. Offer food that is simple to digest and prepare in a way that keeps the nutrients. Fruits and vegetables are essential because they provide the roughage needed for the digestive system to function and avoid constipation. Steer clear of more fibrous vegetables to prevent irritation of the tract. Until the problem is treated, all fibrous substances must be avoided in instances of diarrhea.

You shouldn't serve invalid meals if you have a cold, a cough, or any other contagious ailment. For serving meals, utensils, plates, cutlery, and tray cloths should be clean.

Meals for the sick or recovering should be provided often. Once it comes time for dinner, patients shouldn't be kept waiting.

Before eating, the sick or disabled person should feel comfortable.

Some Recommendations For Ill And Recuperating Patients.

1. Any beverage or milk flavored with Ovaltine.

2. A barely cooked egg.
3. MoinMoin with pap, a bean pudding.
4. Vegetable, Fish, or meat soups.
5. Mashyam, cocoyam, and potato cassava
6. Milk pudding with fresh juice and custard.

CHAPTER 5

VEGETARIAN COOKING

A person who abstains from eating meat, Fish, and sometimes animal products—particularly for ethical, spiritual, or health reasons is a vegetarian

People who avoid eating the byproducts or results of animal slaughter are known as vegetarians. The following foods are off-limits to vegetarians: Fish, shellfish, insects, rennet, gelatin, and other forms of animal protein stock or fats derived from animal slaughter—meat, such as beef, hog, and game.

several vegetarian dietary options. These consist of:

Lacto-ovo-vegetarian. This diet forgoes all forms of meat and Fish but includes dairy products and eggs.

Lacto-vegetarian. On this diet, dairy products are consumed instead of meat, Fish, or eggs.

Ovo-vegetarian. On this diet, people only eat eggs; they don't eat any meat, Fish, or dairy items.

Pescatarian. The only meats allowed on this diet are Fish and other forms of shellfish.

A vegan diet forgoes all animal products, including honey and dairy, as well as meat, Fish, poultry, eggs, and dairy products.

A predominantly vegetarian diet that sometimes includes meat, Fish, or fowl is known as a **flexitarian diet**.

Essential Ingredients in Vegetarian Cuisine

A varied selection of fruits, vegetables, grains, healthy fats, and proteins should be part of a vegetarian diet. Include a variety of protein-rich plant foods like nuts, seeds, legumes, tempeh, tofu, and seitan in your diet to supplement the protein given by meat.

Calcium

To acquire their recommended daily intake of calcium, vegetarians should eat a range of calcium-rich foods.

Lactose-containing foods are a good source of calcium. Calcium may be gained from plant-based foods if your diet does not contain dairy products, however, the quantity of calcium that the body can absorb from these foods varies.

Here is a list of calcium-rich foods that are suitable for vegetarians:

Milk, yogurt, and cheese with reduced or no fat

Plant-based kinds of milk with added nutrients, such as soy or almond

Prepared foods that have been fortified

enhanced with calcium juice

Cathodic tofu

Several leafy green vegetables, such as kale, collard greens, and turnip greens

Broccoli

Beans, such as black beans, chickpeas, and soybeans

almond butter with almonds.

Iron

To satisfy daily needs, vegetarians should eat a range of iron-rich foods. Every meal should include a source of vitamin C, such as citrus fruits, peppers, or tomatoes, to assist boost iron absorption.

Iron comes from sources like

Fortified morning cereals.

Soybeans

A few dark leafy greens, such as chard and spinach

Beans

Eggs.

Protein

Veggie and animal meals both include protein. If you consume a variety of meals and get enough calories throughout the day, your body will produce adequate complete protein on its own.

Among the vegetarian sources of protein are:

Legumes like lentils, beans, and peas

whole grains

Soy-based goods
nut jars of butter with nuts
dairy goods
Eggs.

Vitamin B12

All meals of animal origin, such as eggs and dairy products, include vitamin B12. Many vegetarians, particularly vegans, may have concerns about getting enough vitamin B12. Any vegetarians should pick vitamin B12-fortified meals and discuss if vitamin B12 (cobalamin) supplements are appropriate for them with their doctor.

Vitamin B12 sources that are vegetarian include:

Foods fortified with vitamin B12, such as ready-to-eat cereals, soy milk, and nutritional yeast (Check the label carefully since not all goods on the market have vitamin B12 fortification.)
dairy goods
Eggs.

Vitamin D

Vitamin D is not naturally present in many foods, but it is added to many dairy products in the US. People who prefer not to consume dairy products and who do not often get exposure to sunshine should speak with their doctor about the need to take a vitamin D supplement.

sources of vitamin D that are vegetarian include:

Eggs

Soy milk, cow's milk, orange juice, and ready-to-eat cereals are all fortified with vitamin D.

UV-light-exposed mushrooms.

Healthy vegetarian eating:

Every day, eat a variety of fruits and vegetables.

Meals should be based on starchy carbs.

Calcium must be obtained via dairy products or substitutes.

Eat eggs, beans, lentils, and other protein-rich foods.

Pick spreads and oils that are unsaturated.
Eat less food that is heavy in fat, salt, and sugar.

Health Benefits

There are many health advantages to following a vegetarian diet.
A vegetarian diet may also benefit your health in several different ways.
It promotes weight loss: If you're trying to lose weight, switching to a vegetarian diet may be helpful. Vegetarian diets were nearly two times more effective than low-calorie diets in reducing body weight.
Vegetarian diets may reduce the risk of cancer.
Blood sugar stabilization: Vegetarian diets may aid in maintaining normal blood sugar levels. By long-term regulating blood sugar levels, vegetarian diets may also help people avoid developing diabetes.
Encourages Heart Health
Meal suggestions for vegetarians
Egg and rice stew
Beans

Custard sauce with fruit salad
Fruit with stew and fried plantains and potatoes

CHAPTER 6

FOOD PRESERVATION

Whether you want to eat the food at home, prepare it in a professional kitchen, or sell it straight to customers, food preservation describes the procedures you employ to get the food ready for secure, long-term storage. Food processing procedures that stops the development of microbes like yeast and reduce the rancidity-causing oxidation of lipids are examples of food preservation. The major reason food is preserved is to prevent decay-related food loss.

Techniques for food preservation

Compared to raw food, preserved food can be kept for a longer time. There are several ways to preserve food. The typical techniques include:

I1. **Freezing**: In this food preservation technique, food is put in a freezer where it swiftly freezes. A temperature of zero degrees Celsius (°C) or below may be required for frozen food of high quality. Meat, seafood, tomatoes, and other foods are a few examples of what may be frozen to preserve food.

2. **Solar or sun drying:** Drying may be accomplished using electricity or the sun's heat. To prevent spoiling, vegetables, maize, beans, cassava chips, yam chips, etc., are preserved by drying.

3. **Smoking**: This technique uses this technique to preserve foods like meat and Fish. It entails laying the Fish or meat over a fire so that the heat and hot smoke from the fire will dry it. Smoking preserves foods like crayfish, smoked Fish, beef, etc.

4. **Canning**: Sardines, sweet corn, baked beans, and other products are prepared in a specific oil

or paste before being packed in airtight cans under stringent sanitary guidelines.

5. **Salting**: This technique is used to preserve meat and Fish from farms. The most used chemical for food preservation is salt. Salt helps food dry quickly and kills microorganisms.

Preservation of Food Is Important

Three factors make food preservation crucial:

Food that has been stored for a long time runs the significant danger of becoming bad from germs like E. coli, Salmonella, and other infections. To quickly proliferate in food, bacteria just require temperature, moisture, and time; however, food preservation blocks one or more of these factors and halts their development.

Since food deteriorates over time due to spoiling, it must be kept at its highest quality. While moderate spoilage often does not render food dangerous to consume, it has a noticeable impact on the meal's flavor, texture, and appearance. The nutritional content of certain foods may also be retained with the aid of proper food preservation.

To reduce waste, which is expensive both at home and in a business environment. While it's best to refrain from purchasing more food than you can use, some safe preservation techniques may help you store produce like fruits, meat, and vegetables far beyond their specific expiry date.

CONCLUSION

Four criteria must be met for good, healthy food. Dieters should steer clear of unhealthy and unappealing meals.

The brain and hormones, among other parts of the body, are severely harmed by poor, unhealthy nutrition. Food that is bad for you should be eliminated from your life and avoided wherever feasibly.

One of the worst effects of a poor diet is inflammation, which is the root of many diseases. Although it is possible to believe that these problems are primarily a result of heredity, this is untrue.

The majority of seed oils, sugars, treats, cereals, beans, and dairy products are bad for your health. These foods must be avoided for health reasons.

The body benefits from eating meat from suitable sources, vegetables, eggs, and fruits, as well as certain fats. They should comprise the majority of the diet.

As long as dieters follow basic guidelines, adhere to flexible portion size restrictions, and ensure the right combination of food groups is on the plate, meal planning may be simple. Those may be modified based on a person's body type.

A dieter will see significant improvements in their well-being if they cut out the poor meals and stick to good foods for 30 days.

www.ingramcontent.com/pod-product-compliance
Lightning Source LLC
LaVergne TN
LVHW041251150826
845673LV00008B/2541

* 9 7 9 8 3 5 6 8 4 0 3 1 9 *